Choosing:
A
Healthy
Lifestyle

("Change")

Book
2

By Jeff Shammah

Alphabet

We learn the letters of the alphabet as our foundation in creating words, sentences, paragraphs, and stories. Allowing us to speak, read, write, and communicate.

The books on "Exercise" and now the new series Choosing: A Healthy Lifestyle, are being written from **basic understanding ("Exercise"),** to **advance application.** In order to help **"you"** as an individual, achieve **"A Healthy Lifestyle".**

1. No Table of Contents–**purposefully done,** in order to **discourage** skipping ahead to one's interest or favorite topic.

2. Written in **small bites,** over time, in order to **encourage** full comprehension and **holistic** (whole) **digestion** of information.

3. Because, reaching one's **full potential,** is dependent upon learning proper basics. As my teacher would say:

"Your basics are your advance, your advance are your basics."

Universal Principle

"Change"

Growth requires change,
and change can illicit
feelings of :

Fear, Anxiety
and Discomfort (pain).

Discipline helps us overcome fear, anxiety, and discomfort. In order to achieve **growth**.

How do we practice **discipline?**

By **"actively"** living it. Not, just reading, writing or speaking about it. But the **active** act of **physically** doing it through **exercise** (practice).

⭐ The **human body** is like a Ferrari/Lamborghini– it needs to be raced (challenged), at healthy intervals, in order to operate properly. When **mind, body,** and **breath** become **one,** through repetitive **motion** (exercise) and **non-motion** (meditation), it becomes:

Discipline

Meditation, both motion (physical) and motionless (stillness), helps unite the **mind, body,** and **breath** (spirit).

Spirituality is a by product of a holistic approach (well rounded). Allowing us to reach our full potential as individuals.

Results

How do we know if what we are doing is working?

Results are achieved through the application of **universal principles** over time:

Hard work (correctly applied), **diligence** (consistency), and **patience** (time).

Universal principles work in **all** situations, **not,** just our favorite; and they **adapt** and **change** as we change:

Single • Married • Divorced

Employed • Unemployed • Retired

Children • No children

Healthy • Unhealthy

Happy • Unhappy, etc.

If the body actually spoke verbally, rather than through signs and symptoms, it would say:

> "I have been there for you...
> *can you please,*
> now be there for me?"

Escapism

Fiction • Romance • Mystery

How about escaping into **your own life,** instead of away from your life?

Creating your own narrative through choosing a healthy lifestyle, that leads to **romance** and **mystery.** Through the use of your **imagination,** in order to create **your best life.**

Figuring out what needs to change, and how to go about doing it, can be quite challenging. Starting with your health, and choosing the right exercises at the right time in your life, will be the key to your success.

"Feel-good hormones" are what **exercising**

triggers the release of in your brain and throughout your body (nervous system). As far as our current understanding (science):

Endorphins: the brain's "natural painkiller" can help

improve your mood and reduce stress (debated as to whether it crosses the blood-brain barrier).

Endocannabinoids: able to cross the blood-brain

barrier. Associated with reduced anxiety and promoting feelings of calm.

Dopamine: (neurotransmitter) released by the brain

as part of a rewards system, associated with pleasure and motivation.

Seratonin: (neurotransmitter) helps regulate mood and support sleep, appetite, and digestion (cool down period).

Exercise has an anti depressive effect on the mind and body. The Hippocampus, part of the brain associated with memory and learning. May increase in volume and improved function, through regular exercise.

> We cannot and should
> not escape
> *our human nature,*
> *our primal selves.*

Exercising (indoors/outdoors) can take the place of our hunter gatherer ancestry. Satisfying our nature to hunt, gather, and consume (eat). But; in a healthy, civilized, and respectful (to nature) manner. In order to calm the "savage beast" within us. As opposed to the boredom and regression that sets in and consumes us, when we don't have a **healthy outlet** for our emotions:

Music: Listening, playing, composing

Dance: Self expression

Nature: Outdoor activities

Art: Physical manifestation

Exercise: Physical exertion and sweat

When we do not practice a healthy form of release
(outlet), it forms the basis for **future aging health issues.**
A **mind** and **body** being affected by **lifestyle choices,**
progressing slowly over time (decades), to the point where:

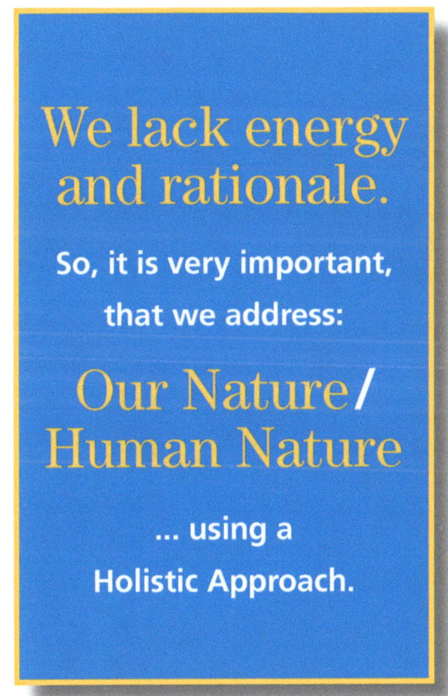

What is a
Holistic Approach

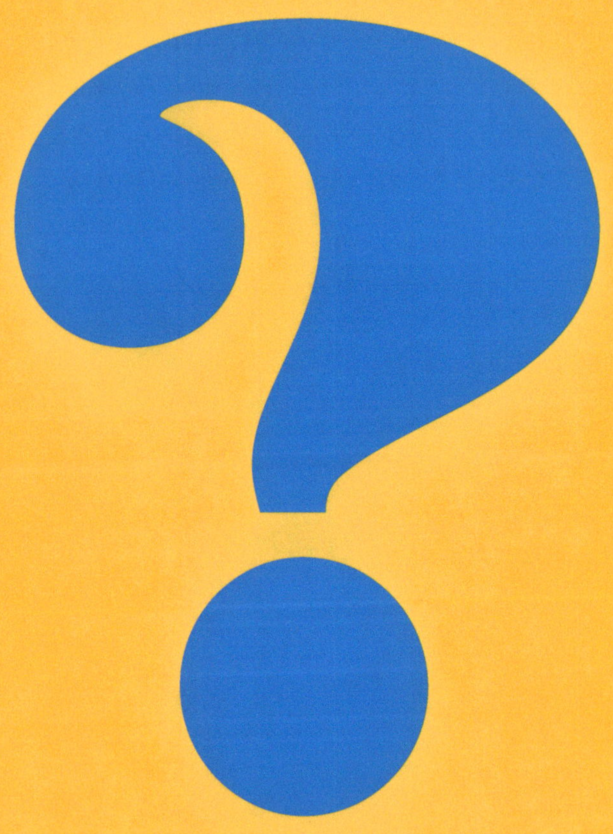

Means to **stop** relying on one thing (favorite), to fix all things (dislikes). We need to practice **balance** (likes and dislikes), in order to achieve Mental, Emotional, and Physical equilibrium (homeostasis).

Proper exercise and training in any discipline (program), should help us **throughout our lives, not** just in the moment (fad diets and extreme exercises). Basic principles that are universal, and applied to **all forms** of exercise and health, therefore **holistic.**

Holistic health is like the S&P 500 (stock market index). A diversified approach that makes steady consistent progress over time. Avoiding, when possible, extreme reactions to volatility (ups and downs of life). Ultimately ending higher (healthier), with more gains than losses. Paying **dividends**–the sooner you start investing in your health, the sooner you will start receiving dividends (improvements and gains.)

Do not rely

on any one thing to make up for, or cover, everything.
A little bit of all (holisticity), will lead to a:

Sum Total

that is **greater** and more **balanced.**

Everything comes down to security and insecurity **(fear).**
A holistic (balanced) approach relieves **fear** and **prejudice,**
and encourages open-mindedness. Leading to **harmony.**

> Being at peace
> with oneself, *and*
> *accepting* that we
> will *never* be in
> complete control.

Holisticity in practice

Have you ever read a book where you were inspired by the lead character (protagonist) and it read "they were born, everything went great, and they died"?

No, it was the adventures and the obstacles, that they overcame, that inspired us. In a book, this takes place over several pages and chapters. But, in real life, it took **years.**

Time,
and our use of it, is our greatest challenge.

A HOLISTIC APPROACH IS LIKE LIFE, IT IS:

ALL ENCOMPASSING!

"Change"

Repetition

Once, we are **aware** of the need for change. It is followed by the *Why? How?* and *What? (Books 1, 2 and 3 of the Exercise series).*

When that is established through the help and guidance of a Doctor, Therapist, Personal Trainer, Nutritionist etc.

The real work begins!

Practice, is a form of **repetition.** The consistent, progressive, and patient performance of your exercise routine, through trial and error. Slowly leading towards **your Individual Health Prescription. Not, one-size-fits all. Long term results, not, short-term** (momentary) **results.**

Mindfully–only correct practice leads towards improvement *(Book 1 of the Exercise series)*

> *Practice*
> does not make
> *perfect.*

*You don't memorize life,
you live it!*

And as you gain **experience,** you refer back to it, in order to
guide your **future decisions.** Otherwise, there is no **wisdom.**
(Book 1 of the Exercise series)

*Wisdom is the
proper use of experience.*

Breath/Oxygen

The first and most important nutrient for the Human Body is **Oxygen** (O_2). **Breath** (breathing) is the tool that **unifies** the **mind** and **body,** helping us to achieve **balance.**

During times of excitement, fear, and stress, it is elevated (sympathetic), fight or flight. During times of relaxation and digestion, it is slower (parasympathetic), allowing us to recuperate. These two branches (sympathetic/parasympathetic) are part of our Autonomic Nervous System.

Exercise, allows us to practice and improve our breathing and command of these two. Leading towards a state of homeostasis (balance), and eventually, maybe, even meditation.

Whether you become aware of the **need** to improve your breathing and oxygen consumption (VO_2 max) for:

- Asthma, COPD, Emphysema, etc.
- Improved exercise performance
- Giving birth
- Singing, acting
- Digestion
- Aging, etc.

> ## It is oxygen,
> ### *the life force (electricity)*
> ## that powers life.

Kung-Fu, Yoga, Cardio, Strength Training, Free Diving, Boxing, MMA, Running, Rock Climbing, etc. **all** have proven, time tested techniques, to improve our usage and control of **oxygen** (breath). In order to help us improve our **health** and **performance.**

There is **no, one correct way to breathe.** It depends on the **situation, ailment, technique** or **system.**

⭐ It is necessary, to have proper guidance and instruction. From your Doctor, or accredited teacher in your chosen discipline (system/class). In order to learn how to improve your breathing.

Core

...as it relates to the use of muscles while exercising. Is a **location** found at the **center** of the Human Body. Composed of various muscles of the abdominal, lower back, and buttocks area. It is the **foundation** *(Book 2 of Exercise series)* of physical movement (locomotion) when exercising and participating in sports and activities. When properly utilized through both **strength** and **flexibility,** can also help improve problems with:

- Sciatica
- Bladder control
- Sexual function
- Posture

It does not belong to a class, title, or system. **All forms** of healthy and proper movement should initiate from your **Core** (center). Directed by your brain and provide **power** and **strength** to the **lower** and **upper body.**

This means that **"everyone"** will benefit from **young** to **older, layperson** to **athlete.** In learning how to recognize, strengthen, and use their **core muscles.**

So, **do not** allow yourself to be **misled** into thinking that only "this class" or "that system" (marketing), teaches proper use of the core. **All** classes and **all** systems **when properly taught.** Should, and will, teach us about the proper use and importance, of core muscles.

This is wonderful, and gives us **hope.** That we can **all** find **"a way"** to exercise, that works best for our **individual character** and **individual needs.**

There is no
one size fits all.

Endurance

...that is what a **long happy life** requires. **Happiness,** is **not a possession,** it is something we **practice.** A state of being, that comes and goes, depending upon our circumstances.

How are we to withstand life's many challenges, over a **long period** of time, without **physical, mental** and **emotional, endurance?**

The **concept of aging,** is all relative to the **individual.** The 30 year old says to the 20 year old *"wait til you get to my age."* The 40 year old says to the 30 year old *"that's nothing, wait until you're my age."* The 50 year old says *"you'll see, it all changes once you turn 50."* This goes on and on, until the 90 year old says *"you are all kids, I would love to be your age again!"*

We waste three quarters of our lives, complaining about how no one understands us. Why should they? When we often, do not even understand ourselves.

Show them,
or better yet,
show yourself!

By instead, choosing to live, **your best life:**

"In the moment"

(Book 2 Exercise series)

*"Tomorrow
is promised to no one"*

When we focus on, and do our best, in the **present** moment,
we will have:

Less regrets–what living in the **past** is.

A brighter future–what **"Hope"** is all about.

By practicing the art of living in the moment. We will have less regrets and more pleasant memories. Knowing that we did our best at the time. We will have set ourselves up for a brighter future, by **not,** wasting the time we had to do so. We will ultimately experience **less fear,** because living in fear is about regretting the **past,** and being afraid of the **future.**

How do we **"practice" the art of living in the present?**

Self Awareness...

> If we do not recognize the
> *need for change,*
> we will not be willing to do
> the *work* necessary,
> in order to *achieve* it!

"Change" in Action!

Good Morning...

is preceded by a good night's **sleep** *(Book 1 of Choosing a Healthy Lifestyle).*

Generally 6–9 hours of sleep dependent on the individual. With the goal of achieving regular sleeping patterns (times) of going to bed, and awakening. As we age, our intervals will change, as to whether we sleep continuously, in parts, or use daily naps. What matters most is that **you feel rested. Not,** an exact number for all people.

⭐ Illness (mental, emotional, and physical), and parent's of new born babies, will find this a challenge, if not impossible (work with your doctor). Prioritize addressing this (sleep), in your **new** health routine.

1st Leave Time

Refrain from getting up late and rushing around.

2nd Water

The Human Body awakens from a good night's sleep in a state of **dehydration.** 1–2 glasses (8–16 oz) of water **before breakfast** and **coffee,** is **crucial** to restoring your body's **hydration.** From the internal processes (work) that were going on, while you were sleeping *(Book 1-Choosing a Healthy Lifestyle).*

Avoid starting your day with coffee, especially **not,** on an empty stomach. The corrosive (damaging) effects of the acid on the lining of your stomach (empty–without breakfast), over time, is potentially dangerous to your health.

3rd Exercise, Stretching and Meditation

(30–45 minutes)

Morning's are a great time to exercise and meditate before the day's work, responsibilities, and surprises, get in the way.

★ You will need to learn and decide, as to whether to have breakfast first (leaving time for digestion) one hour before or to eat afterwards. Depending upon the previous night's dinner time, and your tolerance for morning meals.

Whether at home, in a class, or outside. Making time in the morning to exercise and start your day with the sunrise, allows you to maintain harmony (circadian rhythm) with nature; and helps achieve mental, emotional, and physical **clarity.**

4th Breakfast

(30–45 minutes)

Avoid skipping breakfast, or starting your day with junk food (doughnuts, pastries). Regardless of whether you are a breakfast eater or not, or the amount of food you choose to eat. Work on, and practice, having something nutritious (vitamins and minerals) to start your day. That includes complex carbohydrates, healthy fats, and protein (plant/animal).

- **Greek yogurt** (unsweetened) add nuts and fruit separately.

- **Oatmeal** (whole oats and grains) unsweetened, adding nuts and fruit separately.

- **Whole grain, multi-grain cereals** and **breads** (low in sodium and sugar).

- **Eggs** (1–2) preferably whole (to provide more vitamins and minerals) or egg whites.

- **Meats** or **plant based protein:** turkey, pork, liver, tempeh, tofu, beans, etc. (unprocessed, grass fed, lean, and organic).

- **Fish** (wild caught or sustainable) salmon, mackerel, trout, sardines, etc.

- **Healthy fats:** olive oil, avocado, flaxseed, sesame, etc.

- **Whole Milk** (8oz): a glass of whole milk contains your carbohydrates, fats and protein in one cup.

Always aware of your individual allergies and intolerances.

Good Afternoon…

also, a wonderful time to exercise, stretch, meditate, and have a nutritious meal.

⭐ **If working, your routine will need to be clear, concise (short), and purposeful (intention). Know what it is you need to do, and do it. Time is of the essence.**

Your exercise routine will take 15–30 minutes. Leaving 30–45 minutes for eating. Your lunch needs to be pre-planned or prepared. Also, including complex carbohydrates, healthy fats, and protein (plant/animal). Preferably, more time is needed to complete these two. But, in the increasingly fast paced environment that we live in, **most people, will not,** have more time **(reality).**

This is when most individuals "hit a wall" (lethargy). A healthy balanced lunch, **not** junk food or drugs, is a better or healthier answer.

Examples (small or large):

• **Plain yogurt** (unsweetened) add fruits and nuts.

• **Fish, chicken, turkey, etc.**

• **Vegetables, mixed greens**

• **Tofu, tempeh, beans, etc.**

• **A Shake (drink)** fruits and vegetables.

• **Dark chocolate** (70%)

• **Water**

These foods and others like them, will have a positive effect on your energy levels (glycemic index).

⭐ Napping: for others who are older, sleep less hours at night, retired, or have more time on their hands, napping may be an option. In general, early midday (20–45 minute) naps, allow for a refreshed feeling (alertness), without interfering with your bedtime sleep.

(Consult your doctor or sleep specialist)

Good Evening...

When we as "Human Beings" develop regular pattern's of awakening and preparing ourselves with sunrise:

- Leaving time (not rushing) 1–2 hours
- Exercise, stretching, meditation (15–45 minutes)
- Nutritious breakfast (30–45 minutes)

and practice regular lunchtime behaviors:

- Exercise, stretching, meditation
- Nutritious meal (30–45 minutes)

> We are setting
> ourselves up for
> *a Good Evening.*

Exercising in the early evening, is also an option, for those whose mornings and afternoons are impractical. These sessions also need to be clear, concise, and purposeful (30 minutes–1 hour). Due to fatigue from the day's work, and the need to **not** overstimulate yourself. So you do not negatively affect your bedtime.

Your evening meal should also be composed of complex carbohydrates, healthy fats, and proteins (plant/animal).

Examples (small or large):

- **2–3 different types of vegetables** (colors), and or **mixed greens.**

- **Chicken, turkey, fish, tofu, tempeh, beans, etc.** (3–5 oz), (grass fed, wild caught, sustainable, organic, non-processed)

- **Healthy fats** (monounsaturated and polyunsaturated fats) found in foods like olives, avocados, nuts, seeds, and fatty fish.

⭐ Finish your meal (1–3 hours) before your regular bedtime. Those who suffer from **G.E.R.D.** (acid reflux) will benefit from a longer interval between their last meal, and going to bed.

• **Refrain** from exposing yourself to Technological Devices (1–2 hours) before bedtime.

• Create an **ambiance** (environment) and **routine** that prepares you for sleeping (showering, face washing, teeth brushing, etc.) Darkening the rooms (lights and shades) 1–2 hours before bedtime.

• Watch TV in a different room (not bedroom) when possible, or read in bed (book, not device). So the Body and Mind, see the bedroom as a place for sleep, lovemaking, soothing music, preferably **not** television.

⭐ For those who work the **Night Shift.** You will also benefit from a regular routine and intervals (times) of going to sleep, breakfast, lunch, and dinner. It's just that yours will be the opposite of a daytime worker. Often, **artists** and **creative individuals** tend to function best under these conditions (evening hours).

When, and if, you are able to establish regular, healthy, patterns and cycles of behavior (excluding emergencies):

"You" will have chosen to live, a healthier lifestyle.

And, you will experience a:

Good *morning...*
Good *afternoon... and*
Good *night!*

Misconceptions

Cosmetic/ Non-Cosmetic Muscles

In the "mid-1980's" when I worked for Health Clubs. A common sight was to see an individual looking at themselves in the mirror and obsessing on, and overworking, the muscles that they saw in the front of their body **(cosmetic).** The front of their shoulders, chest muscles, biceps, abdominal muscles, front of their thighs, etc. This has gone on in the past, and continues on to the present day.

But, it is even **more important** to strengthen and increase the flexibility of the muscles, **you do not see** looking back at you in the mirror **(non-cosmetic).**

For they are responsible for holding us upright **(posture),** and moving us around **(locomotion).**

The muscles of your:

• Buttocks

(gluteus maximus, medius, and minimus) exercises:
glute bridges, squats, lunges, pliés, leg raises, donkey kicks, etc.

• Hamstrings

(biceps femoris, semitendinosus, semimembranosis) exercises:
dead lifts, squats, lunges, leg curls, pliés, leg kicks, etc.

• Lower-back (to middle)

(erector spinae, multifidus, quadratus lumborum) exercises:
airplane, swimmer, superman, planks, etc.

• Upper-back (middle to upper)

(latissimus dorsi, rhomboids, levator scapulae, trapezius)
exercises:
lat pull downs, pull ups, chin ups, rows, shrugs, etc.

• Calves

(gastrocnemius, soleus, plantaris) exercises:
standing, one leg, and seated calf raises

★ Choose from these exercises according to the health of your joints. Proper form and guidance from your physical therapist, personal trainer, or accredited class instructor is necessary.

Each of these muscles or muscle groups, serves a distinct function. When properly used, **both strength** and **flexibility,** will provide us with improved:

- **Hip:** strength, stability and flexibility
- **Back:** spinal support, strength, stability, and flexibility
- **Improved posture**
- **Balance**
- **Coordination**
- **Extension:** abduction, adduction and rotation.

On your quest to leading a healthier life through exercising. Pay **more attention** to what you do not see, **non-cosmetic muscles.** For these muscles will serve you best throughout your life, whether:

- General health
- Athletic health
- Aging

> *"It's what you* don't see,
> *that catches up with you."*

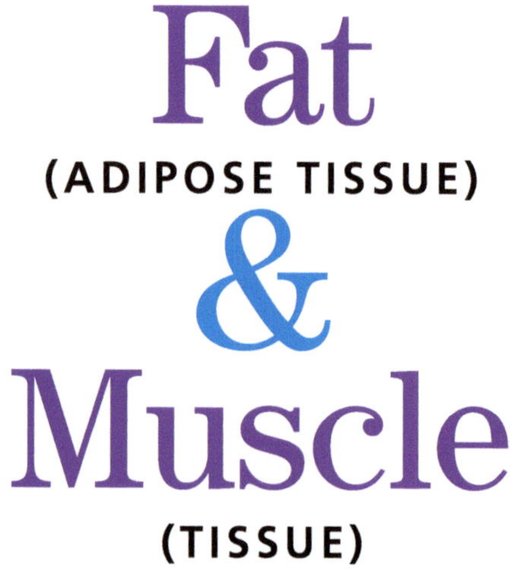

Fat
(ADIPOSE TISSUE)
&
Muscle
(TISSUE)

Fat and Muscle are made up of **very different properties.**

One cannot turn into the other!

They are composed of different cell structures, carry out different functions in the body, have different metabolic rates, and different densities.

Both muscle and fat
are needed for a healthy body.

Fat:

- Stores energy for use
- Insulates the body
- Cushions internal organs
- Is less dense (occupies **more** space)
- Has a slower metabolic rate
- Endocrine system (produces and releases hormones that
regulate metabolism, reproduction, and other bodily functions.

Risks associated with high body fat:

- Insulin resistance (type 2 diabetes)
- Cardiovascular disease
- Chronic inflammation
- High blood pressure
- Respiratory problems
- Fertility problems

Muscle:

- Enables movement
- Provides stability
- Denser and compact (occupies **less** space)
- Higher metabolic rate

Benefits of muscle mass:

- Increased strength, fitness, performance
- Joint support (mobility)
- Reduced risk of injury (falling)
- Improved **posture** (support)
- Higher metabolism (24/7)
- Improved immunity (prevention)
- More energy

When one chooses to live a healthier lifestyle, and engages in regular exercise, they will improve their **body composition.** The **ratio of fat, muscle, bone** and **water.**

Increasing the amount of their body weight that is composed of: muscle, bone and tissue.

While...

Decreasing the amount of their body weight that is composed of fat.

Water being affected by:
- Age
- Sex (male or female)
- Consumption (how much you drink)
- Body fat (lean tissue has a higher water content than fat tissue).

★ STRESS ★

Chronic stress can release the hormone **Cortisol,** which can result in:

- Increased appetite and cravings for sugary and fatty foods.
- Increased **fat storage** (visceral fat) surrounding your internal organs (potentially dangerous).
- Insulin sensitivity (high blood sugar)
- Poor sleep

so, through proper:

- Exercise (strength and cardio)
- Nutrition
- Water consumption
- Sleep
- and reduced stress

We will increase muscle while reducing fat. Not, turn fat into muscle.

Metabolism, Nutrition & Exercise

Breakfast, **raises your metabolic rate** (metabolism) through the process of **digestion** (3–5 hours). Skipping it, maintains a **lower metabolic rate.** Since there is nothing to digest, your system operates at a slower rate.

Maintaining this habit throughout your life, teaches the body to "store fat" (like a squirrel hides nuts in winter), in order to operate through the morning hours. Which slowly, over time, contributes to "fat deposits" (adipose tissue) on your body. Usually the abdomen for men, and the hips, back of upper arms, and later the abdomen (menopause), for women.

Cardio (aerobic exercise)–raises your metabolism **momentarily,** for the time (duration) that you are exercising, and a bit afterwards. But, it will then return to your normal rate.

Strength Training–increasing muscle, your body composed of **more muscle, bone** and **tissue,** and **less fat,** improved **body composition. Will raise your metabolism,** 24 hours a day, 7 days a week.

We need **all of the above.**
Nutrition (breakfast), cardio (aerobic exercise),
and strength training.

not, a fad diet

which is *only temporary,* and will lead to *greater weight gain later.*

⭐ **Nutrition Plans**–special note on sharing same meals.
Be careful to **not,** prepare, order or eat, the **same** meals (diet plan) as your partner. **One-size-does not fit all.**
Your individual nutritional needs should take precedence, over the convenience of same meal diet plans.
Take the time, to learn about and eat, **according to your individual needs** and **deficiencies.**

Inflammation

Your **immune system** is your body's **Doctor.** But, it is often **not** working properly or efficiently. *(Book 1 of Exercise series- Human Body "machine of forgiveness").*

Acute Inflammation–the initial reaction by the body, is a **beneficial** response by the immune system. But when this response persists over long periods of time and becomes **Chronic Inflammation,** it then becomes potentially harmful to the Human Body.

Positive reasons for **Acute Inflammation:**
- Healing, cuts, sprains, bruises, etc.
- Recovery from a strenuous workout
- Helping to prevent infection

Negative outcomes of **Chronic Inflammation:**
- Arthritis, (rheumatoid/osteoarthritis, etc.)
- Cancers
- Heart Disease
- Alzheimer's Disease
- Chronic Fatigue Syndromes

Overeating,
Overworking
Overtraining

are all **stresses** on the body that contribute to overuse and repetitive use syndromes *(Athletes-Book 1 of Exercise series)*.

Which may also result in:

Chronic Inflammation (negative inflammation). Potentially leading towards **chronic illness** as we age.

Aging

is relative to **not** just your **genetics,** but also, **how you live.** The amount of **wear** and **tear** you are subjected to throughout your **life.**

Stress plays a major role on how we age, and the quality of our years. There is the kind of stress that leads to **positive change:**

Exercise + Nutrition + Sleep = Results
(stress and adaptation) = (positive change)
(Recuperation-Book 1 of Exercise series)

And there is the kind of stress that leads to **negative change:**

• **Overexercising:** overuse and repetitive use injuries, and future arthritic conditions.
• **Overworking:** Chronic fatigue syndromes, nervous break-downs, autoimmune illnesses.
• **Over** and **under eating:** Obesity, Type 2 Diabetes, Anorexia and Bulimia. *(Nutrition medicine: Book 3 of Exercise Series)*

- **Alcohol** and **Drug Abuse:** high blood pressure, heart disease, stroke, liver disease, digestive problems, psychological problems, and cancers.

Examples:

Athletes will subject their body's to **more stress** (high risk) in a short period of time (5–25 years), than most in a **lifetime.** Experiencing chronic pains and discomforts:

- Arthritis, bursitis, tendinitis, etc.
- Surgeries

by middle age (40–60 years), that would normally take affect during older age (70–90 years).

High Stress Jobs:

- Parenting
- President, CEO
- Police Officer, Fireman
- Doctors, nurses, therapists, teachers
- Stockbroker, lawyer, etc.

Leading towards:

- Depression
- Chronic fatigue syndromes
- Autoimmune illnesses
- Nervous breakdowns

also, sooner, rather than later.

For many of the **less fortunate** there is **no easy answer** or **fix:**

- Poverty
- Prejudice
- Hunger and malnutrition
- War
- Genetic disease or illness

For others who are **more fortunate:**

- Education
- Employment
- Nutritious food and clean water
- Loving family

It comes down to a choice:

How do we wish to live our lives?
Why do we need to exercise?

Because,

everything in life requires health!

Health *is both a* necessity *and a luxury.*

Acknowledgment

Why do I advocate (recommend), all healthy forms of **exercise** and **art?**

Because, when done properly, they **all** work, and can improve our health.

My over 40 years of experience as a personal trainer and business owner. With 25 of those years renting space to, and exchanging services with, freelance health professionals of different exercise and therapeutic arts. Has taught me, so far, that there are good teachers and not so good teachers, in **all forms** of **exercise, arts,** and **systems.**

Do not, assume "magical qualities" touted by marketing.

Instead,

Choose to be smart...
Believe in yourself...
Make changes when necessary...

and...

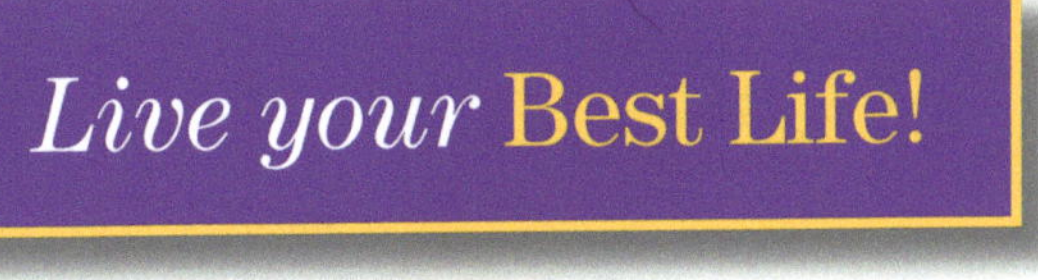

To be
continued...

Credits

Photography
Susie Lang

Design
Jeffrey Shammah with Gloria Gregurovich